Marvelous Messages
from Your Body

Use the Meaning of an Ailment
to Guide Your Life

Jamie Linn Saloff

SENT
BOOKS

**SENT
BOOKS**

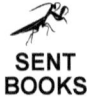

Sent Books
P. O. Box 339
Edinboro, PA, 16412

Cover image adapted from Artant and Lumezia/iStockPhoto.com. Used
with permission. Body images drawn by M. G. Saloff.

Print: ISBN 978-1-7325300-0-3
Ebook: ISBN 978-1-7325300-3-4
Library of Congress Control Number: 2019908834
First edition, © 2016, Revised edition © 2021-2024. v. 4.0
Copyright information available upon request.

For Timothy

Visit Jamie's website at:
https://www.MarvelousMessages.com

"If medicine is adequate to the curing of disease,
why are chronic diseases so prevalent?"

Andrew Jackson Davis,
The Great Harmonia, Vol I, circa 1850

The main purpose of this book is to show how a physical symptom can be interpreted as a message from your heart and soul.

The message may be a nudge to do that thing you've been putting off, that thing your heart's longing to do.

It might be to remind you how something or someone in your life is detrimental to your soul's sacred path.

You may have a desire to resolve a long-term life situation but fear taking any action, don't know what action to take, or believe a resolution isn't possible.

This book shows a way to acknowledge the message that is uniquely yours, interpret it into an understandable form, and discover the steps offered to you through its message.

When you listen to your body and follow its guidance, your life takes on new meaning and direction. Amazing possibilities are awakened in your life.

Contents

"If I succeed in changing the minds of men
enough to investigate
they will see that disease is what follows an opinion,
and that wisdom that will destroy the opinion
and make the cure.
Then the cure will be attributed to
a superior Wisdom,
not a power...."

"I prophesy that the time will come
when men and women shall heal all manner of diseases
by the words of their mouth."

Phineas Parkhurst Quimby
The Quimby Manuscripts, p. 277 & 286

Is This You?

Have you recently struggled with any of the following?

> ▷ *Physical pain, chronic illness?*

> ▷ *Allergies?*

> ▷ *Recurring injuries?*

> ▷ *Exhaustion from lack of downtime? Sleepless nights?*

> ▷ *Unrest and a feeling that something is missing?*

> ▷ *Overwhelmed? Are you being hit from all sides and from others' calls for help?*

> ▷ *Irritability, quick to snap?*

> ▷ *Doubting yourself when you're normally self-assured?*

> ▷ *Dissatisfaction, frustration, indifference? Stress?*

> ▷ *Depression, crying jags, lack of joy?*

> ▷ *Have you carried an unfulfilled desire that has tugged at your heart for years?*

Pain speaks to me. For many years I've helped others use their aches and pains as a means of rejuvenating their lives. I teach new ways to listen to your body to tap into your internal guidance and follow your heart. If you are nodding yes to items on this list, this guidebook was designed for you.

What Do the Aforementioned Side Effects Indicate?

Your body is a miracle of miracles. It's made up of a host of "computers" working in symphonic harmony to monitor and regulate all your body's core tasks, including your heartbeat, your breathing, your digestive functions, your thought processes, your nervous system, and more. Most amazingly, those "computers" are generated from living, "breathing," growing, changing, interactive cells interconnected and communicating the body's needs through an emotional mind/body network.

The cellular connection part was first brought to the public in the modern era in 1997 by Candice Pert (*Molecules of Emotion*—which took me years to finally pick up and read), and later furthered in 2005 by cellular biologist, Bruce Lipton *(Biology of Belief*—a book whose opening science-based chapters were so hard for me to get through but so worth it.) At last, there lay before me the scientific proof of what I had known all along, our bodies can speak to us about our current and future lives through our pain. (So much more has come forward since!)

When your body is using a symptom to get your attention, it's often because you've blatantly avoided all the other means God (or however you perceive the Divine) attempted in order to move you toward your sacred calling and deepest heart's desires. It's like you got the memo, crumbled it, heard the phone ring, let it go to voicemail, saw the email, deleted it... and now you're here with an achy back, a bad knee, raging allergies, or worse. Sometimes much, much worse.

Even though our healthy body seems very important to us, our soul's sacred mission is first and foremost. The body will do whatever is necessary to preserve and pursue its calling, even if it means sacrificing some physical function or bearing tremendous physical pain.

It seems ridiculous that our body (or God) would allow us to suffer in pain for any reason. It's easier to believe, however wrongly, that our pain is due to some punishment, sin, or bad luck on our part. Yet, when we build emotional blocks that prevent us from reaching our predestined goal, our body devises a way to pull all the blocks down. A symptom can act as a catch valve. The more we push in the wrong direction, the harder the safety catch pulls back.

Think about how a leafy potted plant may begin to drop its leaves in order to preserve its roots. The plant doesn't need it's leaves as much as its roots which provide its sustenance. Our body sometimes acts in that way too.

You are on the threshold of transition.

You've been guided to move forward toward your sacred calling, but for whatever reason, you may have stalled. Maybe the steps you need to take feel too overwhelming or frightening. Maybe you've been afraid of what you might lose (forgetting or not knowing what you might gain). Maybe you just can't see your way forward. You've been so locked into the daily grind and the human rat race that you've lost track of the *you* that you once wanted to become.

You're now being offered encouragement to act. Your physical body is showing you the way. The universe knows when life becomes uncomfortable you will be spurred toward your destined pathway. It might even feel as if the body is saying, *"If you want to do this the hard way, that's fine with me."*

Those who identify and implement their Guided Action Step— discovered by listening to the body's messages—find their lives shift rapidly. The changes experienced in the following weeks happen so quickly, so synchronistically, so naturally, that many forget that it all began here with a few simple exercises.

Many of my clients are able to make major life shifts with long-term results such as:

- ▷ Quit their day job
- ▷ Start a new business
- ▷ Leave a bad relationship
- ▷ Find the love of their life
- ▷ Buy their dream home
- ▷ Obtain greater wellness

Is this a cure for everything? No. But if you're interested in self-discovery and life improvement, then you'll greatly benefit from the messages found within your body's aches, pains, illnesses, and injuries.

Does every symptom have a message? Probably. But I don't recommend analyzing every papercut and splinter. The idea is not to get caught up in our aches and pains but to move past them.

Are ailments and injuries something we bring on ourselves? Some people believe that. What if God just utilizes what's already occurring as a means to bring home a message we've been reluctant to hear?

Ailments can be powerful allies. Through the methods that follow, you will learn how to interpret an ailment and learn its underlying Marvelous Message.™ They can help you:

> ▷ Discover how ailments actually *empower your life* and lead you toward fulfilling your life's purpose and heart's desires.

> ▷ Encourage you to repair hidden emotional pain you have buried deep within and have failed to *release and/or forgive.*

> ▷ *Lead you to persons or situations* that can provide knowledge, experiences, or contacts you need to fulfill your purpose or goals.

> ▷ Gain understanding of your *underlying obstacles* and how to overcome them.

If you're ready to take some bold steps and create clarity from discomfort, read on. . .

"By interior perception, I discover that
the hundreds of diseases which physicians
have distinguished by as many names,
are simply but Symptoms Of One Disease;
and that this One Disease is caused or created by
a constitutional disturbance in
the circulation of the spiritual principle."

"Toothache, headache, backache—
pain in the heart—
pain in the face—
pain in the chest—
pain in the side—
pain in the limbs—

these are evidences of the spiritual disturbance."

Andrew Jackson Davis,
The Great Harmonia, Vol I, circa 1850

Warning!

This process is designed to quickly reveal and release emotional blocks. If you're not serious about removing the emotionally-charged baggage standing between you and your greatest desires, do not do these exercises! (This is not a joke!)

Some people seriously don't want to "go there." They don't want to revisit certain events from their past. **They do not want to be "triggered."** If this is you, avoid these exercises.

Disclaimer
The author of this book does not dispense medical advice or prescribe the use of any technique as a form of treatment for physical, emotional, or medical problems without the advice of a physician, either directly or indirectly. The intent of the author is only to offer information of a general nature to help you in your quest for personal development and spiritual well-being. In the event you use any of the information in this book for yourself, the author and publisher assume no responsibility for your actions. As always, use common sense when contemplating the exercises in this book.

"When I cure,
there is one disease the less;
but not so when others cure,
for the supply of sickness shows that
there is more disease on hand than there ever was."

"Therefore, the labor for health is slow,
and the manufacture of disease is greater.
The newspapers teem with advertisements of remedies,
showing that the supply of disease increases."

"My theory teaches man to manufacture health;
and, when people go into this occupation,
disease will diminish,
and those who furnish disease and death
will be few and scarce."

Phineas Parkhurst Quimby,
The Quimby Manuscripts, circa 1859

Before You Begin

These quick and easy exercises are best completed when you have some quiet time and can contemplate your discovered answers. If your free time is limited, work one exercise per day until complete.

You may want to gather the following supplies:

- ▷ Paper or journal to write down your answers

- ▷ Favorite pen, markers, or highlighter

- ▷ Dictionary (or use an online one)

Consider working with the help of a friend who may be beneficial in discerning insights you're unable to recognize in yourself. However, each individual bases his/her opinions on their own unique experiences. This means even twins who have faced the same life situations may identify different answers.

Always remember to visualize healing in your body at the end of an exercise as **focusing on discomfort can make it worse**. Using whatever method is most natural to you, see the symptom as being healed and corrected. Visualize yourself as wholly well.

Consult with a doctor for necessary medical treatment. The purpose of this book is intended purely for spiritual enlightenment and personal development. **No treatment or cure is implied.**

Your Healing Mindset

A good friend of mine used to say he knew some people who were *"miserable, and wanted to stay that way."* I'm sure you don't feel that way or you wouldn't be reading this book. Nonetheless, it's important to realize that our healing mindset plays a role in how we receive healing and how we apply it in our lives.

Since God *"sendeth rain on the just and on the unjust,"* we all face challenges in our lives, no matter how honorable we may be. Allow discomfort to serve as an opportunity rather than believing it as an unfortunate incident, fulfillment of karma, or spiteful punishment. I may rely on my physician for necessary treatment, but I use my symptoms as a stepping stone for insights, guidance, and self-growth.

Over twenty years ago, Caroline Myss wrote:

> *So many people are in the midst of a "process" of healing … They are striving to confront their wounds, valiantly working to bring meaning to terrible past experiences and traumas, and exercising compassionate understanding of others who share their wounds. They have redefined their lives around their wounds and accepting them. **They are not working to get beyond their wounds.**** (Emphasis mine.)*

Don't fall prey to a "victim" mentality. Stay steadfast within a positive mindset of healing, and your results will be amazing.

---

*Matthew 5:54, King James Version
**Why People Don't Heal, and How They Can, Caroline Myss, Ph.D.

Let's Get Started!

The first and most important step is to simply assess where you are now in regard to your physical health. Using the diagram on page 14 (or draw your own), create a symptom assessment following the directions and comments below.

Note that a *symptom* is a physical pain, ache, burning, tingling, or other sensation, that you can feel, see, hear, or sense. A symptom is different from a *diagnosis*. A doctor provides a diagnosis that isn't a symptom, but rather a definition for a group of symptoms under a title such as "diabetes," "cancer," "PMS," "high blood pressure," etc. **Leave the diagnoses to your doctor** and focus only on your *symptoms* for this soul-searching body scan.

- ▷ Begin a full-body scan by sitting in a quiet place and taking a few relaxing breaths. Close your eyes and mentally scan your body from the top of your head to the tip of your toes. Don't rush. Carefully contemplate how each part feels and functions. Recognize any areas that aren't optimal.

- ▷ Discover whether or not you can put your finger on the exact spot that you're pinpointing. Sometimes pain isn't where you thought.

- ▷ After you've scanned your body from head to toe, consider what's in your medicine cabinet. Pharmacies are full of creams, lotions, sprays, potions, pills, wraps, tapes, drops, liquids, and a host of other remedies designed to treat your ills. If you're using any of these, there is a symptom involved. Mark it on the chart.

▷ Include eyesight (glasses? contacts?), hearing, teeth and mouth (dental work?). Even if you attribute these to injury, aging, or genetics, these "symptoms" can sometimes offer valuable insights.

▷ Do you have any scars? This permanent mark may carry an ongoing message associated with your Innate Challenges* or soul's mission. A scar's message often evolves over time.

▷ Weight issues,** physical trauma, and life-altering handicaps may apply, but require a more in-depth exploration than is covered here. Like scars, permanent handicaps carry evolving messages, though their reason for existence differs from other symptoms.

▷ Think about the kind of flippant remarks you may say without really thinking about their meaning. *"What a pain in the neck!" "Get off my back!" "He doesn't have a leg to stand on."* These can be clues to messages from your body.

▷ Some clients say they have no symptoms—nothing. Fabulous! I have them place a life issue symbolically in their body and work with that.

---

*See: Appendix: *Innate Challenges*.
**See: Appendix: *Body Image*.

▷ You can also refer to an old injury or childhood illness. When I first explored the meanings hidden in my Hodgkins diagnosis, more than a decade had passed. Yet this self-exploration taught me much about myself, why I had recovered, and how it helped me move forward in my life.

After doing the exercise, it's important to view any symptoms, aches, pains, or symbolic imagery as being healed. **Focusing too much on an ache or pain can actually make it worse.** When you're done with your exploration, visualize healing energies filling your body.

Mark any symptom you are experiencing on this worksheet.
(You can see an example on the next page.)

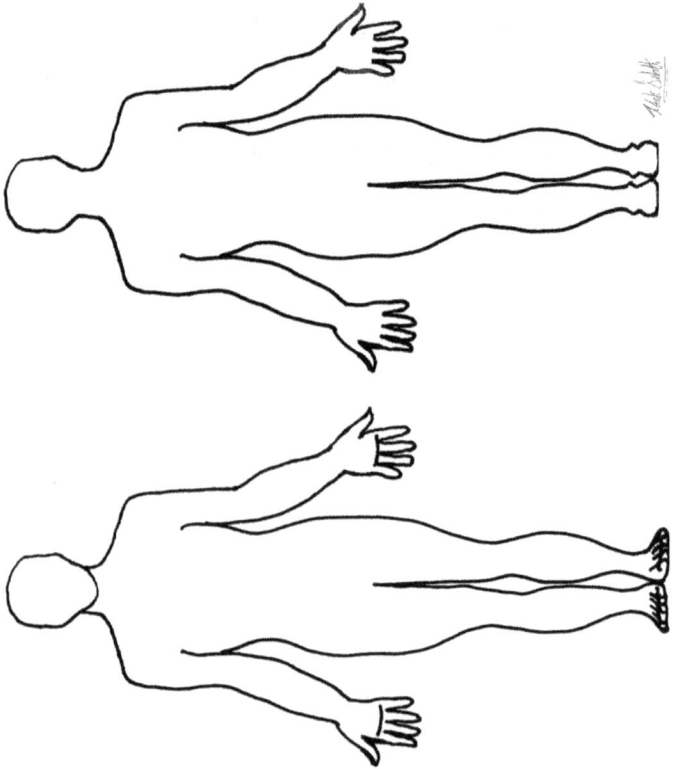

Example. *(I like to draw little symbolic images on mine, but you can use a simple "x" marks the spot.)*

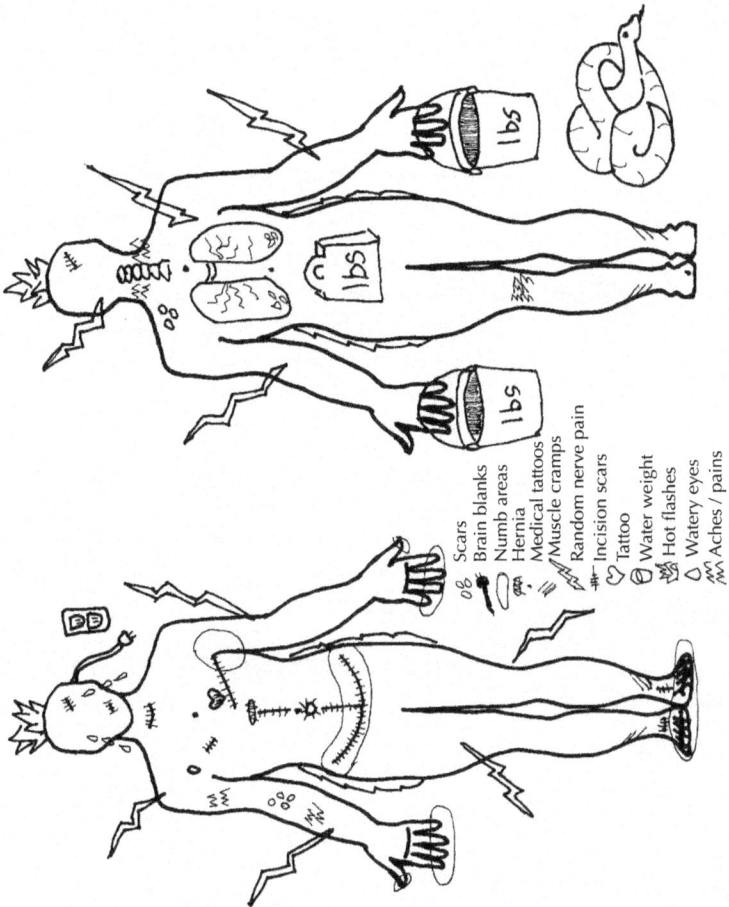

Scars
Brain blanks
Numb areas
Hernia
Medical tattoos
Muscle cramps
Random nerve pain
Incision scars
Tattoo
Water weight
Hot flashes
Watery eyes
Aches / pains

"Humanity is all one vast organization.
When its heart beats
the blood flows to the furthest extremities.
One member can not suffer
without the other members suffering with it.
Unity and sympathy of the parts
constitute the golden chain
which binds the whole together."

"Therefore,
there can be no absolute isolation;
no happiness or misery in the parts,
which the whole does not realize
to some extent."

Andrew Jackson Davis,
The Great Harmonia, Vol. 3, p. 339

Narrowing the Field

Only work with one symptom at a time. I typically ask clients to pick the symptom that is "the most annoying" *right now,* because it's the one trying the hardest to get your attention.

Pick a symptom that is well defined. For example, having body aches "all over" is not as clear as "sinus pain in my right temple" or "joint pain in my left knee."

Don't worry if you are one of those people with LOTS of symptoms. That just means you have many more messages waiting to be heard. And if you're someone with no symptoms—that likely means you're already listening to your inner guidance to some extent. If that's the case, you may gain even more clarity from doing this process.

Scan through your body assessment chart and pick the symptom you want to use for this exercise.

The symptom I will work with is: _____.

Talking to the Mechanic

I refer to the next step as "talking to the mechanic." When our car needs repair, most of us don't know the technical names for the mechanical parts or how they work. We are forced to describe the problem using our own words and frame of reference.

> *"When I start the car, I hear a funny 'whirr, whirr,' and then it 'clunks,' 'sputters,' and backfires."*

Because most of us don't have a medical degree, when we talk to family or friends about our ailments, we usually use our own, made-up language to describe the problem. Our descriptions become colorful stories as we attempt to explain what we are experiencing or how it happened.

Using the symptom you chose on the previous page, pretend you're telling a friend about your discomfort. Commonly, this would be a non-technical language. (If you have medical training, this may be hard for you.) The more you write down, the more you will be able to glean from it as you move forward. **Writing it down is very important**, so please don't skip this step.

Don't try to guess any meanings at this point!

I find this is where most people get tripped up, especially the spiritually minded. They jump ahead to their predetermined meaning losing the best guidance available to them. The next steps are vital in finding the Guided Action Steps you desire.

Write Your Description Here.

Use the box below, or write on your own paper or journal.

Example: *Due to a detached retina, I had surgery on my right eye to prevent the loss of my vision. My eye feels swollen and sore. My vision is blurred and blocked due to trapped fluid and a gas bubble doctors inserted into my eye during surgery. My eye may have been scraped, cut, and stitched. I received a buckle. Later, I received a laser treatment that my doctors compared to being "spot welded." This burned. I experience what I call "searchlights" in my repaired eye. (Full recovery is expected.)*

You're Not Done Yet—There Is More

It's time to dig a little deeper! In order to do so, I am endowing you with two "superpowers"—first, that of having x-ray vision; and second, the ability to reach your hands inside your body.

Using your x-ray vision, look inside your body. Imagine you can see your bones, muscles, tendons, arteries, even cells and fluids. With your "magic" hands, you can move things out of the way or into and out of place. You can zoom in with microscopic vision.

This is when a lot of my clients say, WAIT! What?! I can't do that! I don't know how! To which I say:

> *"Awe, come on! It's just pretend!"*

You don't have to worry about what you see or don't. It's all just make-believe. So give it a try—go inside and look.

Imagine you're along the side of the road, steam billowing from your car's engine. What to do? You might open the hood. Do you know anything about how the motor functions? Not unless you happen to be a mechanic. But you're smart enough to know that a spray of water or a dangling belt means something isn't right. Look inside your body in that same way.

What are you looking for? The cause of the malfunction. *What malfunction?* Something is malfunctioning. If it were working correctly, you wouldn't have pain or discomfort.

"But I don't know what's wrong!"

Come on! You can do this. Trust me. *(Remember, you're just pretending, so you can't do it wrong.)*

Take a few minutes right now to relax, close your eyes, and think about this:

Imagine you're looking inside your body, specifically where you have been experiencing the discomfort. You don't have to explain it technically, eloquently, or medically. Just use your own way to look, see, understand, and explain what you *imagine* is happening. **You can even use a symbolic explanation if that helps, though seeing it anatomically is better.**

With my eye, I imagined the lining part of my eye had become thin and brittle, like old tissue paper. It began to deteriorate. Just like there might be many reasons for tissue paper to age, it might be much the same with the lining of my eye. Maybe I hadn't cared for my vision properly. Maybe it's just a sign of aging.

Keep in mind this is an *imagined* exploration. Your vision might conflict with a doctor's diagnosis. It's okay if what you imagine is different. Just remember it is only an exercise. It's easy to get caught up in a belief. Use the process for its enlightening life insights. Allow your doctors to do the doctoring—that's what their trained to do.

Use the space below to write your imagined "malfunction."

The Ah-ha Dictionary and Your Keywords

Looking at your two descriptions, the "mechanic's story" and your envisioned "x-ray," circle your keywords as follows:

> ▷ Look for words of action, objects (verbs, nouns).
> (My previous example included keywords: *fluid,
> swollen, vision, cut, stitched, welded, burned,
> searchlights,* and *repaired.)*

> ▷ Watch for homonyms, "weight" can also be "wait."

> ▷ Consider tandems, do you think "butter" if
> someone says "bread"?

> ▷ Watch for dual meanings—"acid" can be rock music
> (acid rock); digestive upset (acid reflux); a type of
> rain (acid rain); or an LSD-like drug. Our mind can
> make leaps using word-associations.

> ▷ Note that you may need to look for the core word
> if you wrote down a past-tense version (i.e., "burn"
> not "burned." "Stitch," not "stitched," etc.)

Next, grab a dictionary—or use an online one*. I promise this will be worth the effort! **You are about to discover the deeper, often surprising, messages hidden in your symptom.**

Look up each of your circled keywords. Quickly scan *all* of its definitions. Look *beyond* the meaning of the symptom itself.

------

*I like the WordWeb Dictionary app.

Search instead for phrases that stand out to you as coincidentally relating to *an ongoing life situation*. You should feel an inner reaction or "ping" as you read them. **These are the types of "ah-ha" connections you are looking for.** Write them down!

Let's take a moment to pause here.

No, really. Stop for a moment.

Take a deep breath and let it out.

Even my best of friends glosses over this step.

> *"Yeah, yeah, I already know the meaning of that word."*

> *"Whatever. Let's get to the good part."*

> *"I don't have time to do this right now. I'll do it later."*

Later, never comes. Instead, a few steps from now, you'll find the process doesn't accomplish very much. You won't have the information you need to make the exercise valuable. You might find the whole thing falls flat.

I want you to be amazed at how in tune your body is with what's going on in your life. I want you to be able to recognize how ironically on-target and profound your body's messages are, how unique-to-you they are. If you want that to happen, you have to do all of the steps.

Let's be honest, whether you were gifted this book, paid money for it, or borrowed it, you probably are hoping to get something from reading it. For that to happen, you have to do the following:

▷ Look up your keywords. Look at *all* the definitions.

▷ Consider how *any* of the word's definitions fit your life's situations (usually something currently happening, but occasionally it's from the past).

▷ Write down the key phrases from the words you looked up, most importantly, the ones that gave you that little "ah-ha" "ping" feeling when you read them. (Not every word you look up will do that.)

▷ Maybe you need a better word, one that feels just right. Dr. Eugene T. Gendlin *(Focusing)* explains, when you find the right word, *"There should be a felt response some deep breath inside, some release..."*

▷ Or maybe you need a different dictionary. Sometimes you need to dig deeper into the word's alternative meanings. Often unexpected meanings are found.

For my detached retina example, here's what I found:**

▷ *Detach (ed) - disengage, withdrawal*
▷ *Sore - angry, irked, causing emotional pain or distress*
▷ *Blur (blurry/blurred) - vaguely perceived, confused*

** Definitions from www.Dictionary.com

- ▷ *Block (ed) - obstacle impeding progress; prevent normal function*
- ▷ *Buckle - to give way; yield*
- ▷ *Scraped - to accumulate money by in increments; make one's way with difficulty*

* * *

- ▷ *Fluid - subject to change, available for use; smooth, easy style*
- ▷ *Swollen - expand in size, increase in size or intensity*
- ▷ *Vision - a vivid mental image, especially a fanciful one of the future*
- ▷ *Cut - turn sharply or bypass, reduce in amount, to separate*
- ▷ *Stitched - to fasten or join; to make or mend; unite*
- ▷ *Weld (ed) - to unite or repair closely or intimately*
- ▷ *Burn (ed) - to give off light; to use freely without limits*
- ▷ *Searchlight - used to illuminate or search for distant objects or as a beacon*
- ▷ *Repair - to restore or renew by any process of making good, strengthening, etc.*

Notice that I've organized my list into two sections. The top half seems to echo the essence of happenings in my life pre-surgery. The bottom tends to show a premonition of what's coming post-surgery. (You might not always see your keywords in this way.)

Again, do not form conclusions yet. Just be aware of how the meanings reveal your personal life experience.

Here is what struck a chord with me:

The obvious first—I'd encountered a block. A situation or person may have irked or angered me (anger often covers up underlying hurt), subsequently causing a disconnection (detach) from my heart's desires and life's path. This is a key point to keep in mind as you look at your own keywords.

I'd lost track of my vision (blurred)—not my physical sight, but my hopes/wishes/desires and, ultimately, my highest purpose— my destiny. All I had been striving for was fading away. I'd become distracted, but my body called me back into focus. That's what our bodies do. Looking at my keywords, I can see what this ailment wanted to accomplish.

Thus, my body attempted to create change. Something in my life needed mended (stitched) (repaired) to reunite, renew, or join me back to what I'd pulled away from (detached).

I love that the keywords searchlights and burn (a beacon) and (to give off light; use freely without limits) were telling me this interlude of discomfort was designed to create a realignment so that I might shine brightly (as a soul, a helper, a spirit). This was the best, most encouraging part of the message!

But we are not done yet! There is still more to uncover!

Use this page to write down your important, "ah-ha" key phrases. Note how they connect to your life's situations. Use more paper, if necessary.

A Word of Caution

Even my best friend tries to take the easy way out. In the same way some people prefer to take a pill to mask a symptom rather than discover its cause, my friend will refer to a list book.

What's a list book? It's a reference guide where you look up your symptom—much the same way you might look up a dream symbol—and read its accompanying meaning. If you have a broken leg, you look that up in the book. It tells you what your broken bone means. Some guides are more detailed than others offering long dissertations and often suggesting a meaning stemming from childhood indiscretions, familial abuse, or ingrained negative attitudes. Some offer affirmations, prayers, or healing rituals.

I have twenty-some different list books on my shelves from my days of self-exploration, and here's what I discovered. While I occasionally may find similarities in their answers, none of these offer the same reason for any particular symptom. If there can only be one underlying reason for this problem, why don't all the lists match? Are some of them wrong? Which book(s) has the right answer(s)?

Thus, for my own sake, I created my system to allow me to delve into my psyche, reveal my personal subconscious connections, and help me heal the underlying situations that are hindering my life. It's not as easy as looking at a list. It's often quite a bit more accurate.

Introspection

Recognize how your body is physically manifesting what you are experiencing emotionally in your life. **Think about how intense the situation must be if it's showing up in your physical body.** As you go deeper into the exercise, also consider. . .

> ▷ What situations were taking place in your life at the time this discomfort began? This is the first place to look for your life connections.

> ▷ If you are experiencing multiple symptoms, they often lead to the same life connection. Note that you must explore each symptom on its own. In rare instances, you might glean multiple messages from a singular symptom, though one is usually predominant.

> ▷ Have you seen a recurrence of this symptom with others in your life? (Think: family, friends, coworkers, neighbors, even books, television, or movies you've recently viewed.) *Example:* My father had an amputated leg. Later in life, my new next-door neighbor had an amputated leg.

> ▷ If you cannot find the connection between your current life situations and your symptom, you may need to look further back. Is this the first occurrence? Or have there been others? Work from the time of the first known experience. *Example:*

while exploring my cancer symptoms I realized my
first connection went back nine years pre-diagnosis.

▷ Is this a recurring symptom? When is the first you
remember it? Sometimes they go waaaaay back.
Sit quietly with it and follow the memory threads
backward through time.

Sometimes the malfunction is ridiculously obvious:

I slipped on the ice and broke my leg. . .

I burned my hand on the hot stove. . .

I cut myself while working in the yard. . .

You can then ask yourself:

What else is breaking in my life?

Was I burned by someone; burned out?

How or where have I been cut in my life?

If you know the obvious malfunction, you can move forward
to how it connects to your life, but you must still look up your
definitions from your mechanic's story. They reveal the clues.

Now you're able to create a Guided Action Step to counter the
malfunction mirrored in your life. Taking action tells your body
you're ready to heal (emotionally and physically), and ready to
move forward in life.

Summary

What have you learned so far?

- ▷ Symptoms provide a means to see deeper into your life situations.

- ▷ The words you use to describe your symptoms unveil underlying meanings.

- ▷ When we allow fear, stress, doubt, and indecision to enter our lives, it can reflect back through our physical body.

- ▷ We often first see these messages mirrored in the people around us before we see them within ourselves.* The universe offers an opportunity to learn from them easily before having to fight them off and learn the hard way.

But there is more. . .

---

*See: Appendix: *Mirrors*

The "Fix"

Now that you have visualized a malfunction, it's time to offer yourself a means to mend it. What does this malfunction need? What will make it stop malfunctioning?

Even though this is not a medical diagnosis, trying to "see" and understand the malfunction will help you determine what kind of fix—however imaginary—you need to correct it.

When I'm in session with a client and we reach this juncture, the first thing s/he will typically say to me is:

> *"This is probably going to sound crazy, but what I really want to do is. . ."*

To which I respond: *"That is the perfect place to start!*

However, many of my clients want to gloss over this part. At first, they may be unsure of what to say or create. It sometimes takes some coaxing on my part to get them to dig a little deeper and to be more detailed. It's okay to take some time to do this.

When you are creating your imaginary fix you want to create something that accomplishes the following:

▷ Your fix should heal, remove, repair, and/or prevent any malfunction or damage you've imagined.

▷ Ask yourself, what is causing this and what will stop

it from happening? For example, if you visualize a rash, what is happening in the body that creates this rash? Think about the *result* of the problem *(the rash)* as well as the *cause* of the problem. (How does your body *create* a rash?)

▷ Ask yourself, *"Why is the body doing this? What part of this is protecting the body or helping it heal?"* Then, *"How does the body create this?"* Can you turn the body's action into some action you take in your outer world?

▷ Then ask yourself, *"What will this 'fix' accomplish when complete?"* Or another way would be to ask, *"How would this fix prevent or heal the problem?"* Again, could the answer be used in some way to correct the situation in your life?

▷ Ask yourself the hard questions: What are you able to avoid by having this happen? Who is giving you attention because of this? What does it allow you to say 'no' to? What life changes did this force you to make? Answering honestly will allow you to loosen the symptom's grip and allow you to create an effective countermeasure.

▷ Sometimes the message you receive can be realized as encouragement—and that's a good thing!

Write your fix in this box or on your own paper:

Discovering Your Guided Action Step

This is the fun part! Now all the work you've done so far can pay off in a Guided Action Step that has come directly from deep within you. It's not based on a generic, one-size-fits-all list. It's not all-encompassing. It's a unique-to-you step that helps you get unstuck from a situation you've been struggling with, one you likely recognized when you started digging through your keyword meanings.

Examine your imagined fix and ask yourself:

> *"How can I implement this fix in my life for real?"*

Whoa? What?

At first, you may not see any way that your fix could possibly be made into any real-life action, particularly if you used some wild, imaginary actions for your fix. That's where the thought process comes in. You need to ask yourself,

> *"What is this imaginary fix really accomplishing?"*

From there, you may be able to re-imagine it as a life-action step you could really do.

Sometimes our "fixes" turn out to be funny. My favorite was when I thought I might have a bone spur on my finger. Maybe it was some pre-arthritis. I don't know. I just know that when

I "x-rayed" it with my imaginary vision, I thought of it as "a bone spur." When I began to think of a Guided Action Step, I realized the universe was saying, "Hey, Jamie, we just wanted you to know we are 'spurring' you on to continue doing what you're doing." (Ugh. Okay.) I kept doing what I was doing, and it stopped hurting and disappeared. It hasn't returned.

Check your word choices! I had a neck ache I kept referring to as "out of alignment." This recurring problem went on for quite a while. Nevertheless, I stubbornly kept using the same phrase, "out of alignment," even though I wasn't finding a viable answer. Then one day, I got the idea to change my word to "restricted," and I deciphered a far different, more valuable insight.

Try a different dictionary or a book on etymology or a thesaurus to find alternative meanings for your keywords. You can also look at word choices that pop up in your fix.

Your fix may not seem obvious at first. At times, clients gloss over their fix saying something like, *"I just want to soothe it."* or *"I want to wrap it in a blanket."* Those kinds of fixes don't translate well into a real-world action step. You may need to go back and visualize a more detailed fix.

With my eye issue, I *did* want to soothe it. I wanted to pour something in it or around it that would both heal and comfort it. I felt like it needed protection, a shield of sorts, as if a clear, hard covering would form after this pouring. Of course, this healing liquid would also create clear vision and correction of any problem that might have caused its detachment.

How might this relate to real life and how might I put these steps into action?

Desiring a fix such as "soothing," "comforting," "wrapping it in a blanket," or other similar actions, usually means that your body is simply asking you to "love yourself."

Can you take that in? Can you accept that?

So often, we grumble at our body for any breakdown or pain, we short-change ourselves during times of stress, overwhelm or hardship. We sacrifice ourselves for the sake of helping others, while often regarded as honorable, may not always be the road to our best self. It's okay to love yourself first, then, from that abundance of love within, allow it to flow to others.

For me, the first action step called for was self-love. Others might devise different answers from my keywords, but that is the beauty of this process. We each work it out individually, not based on some pre-determined list.

I realized I also needed to take care of my personal boundaries (thus, the need for a shield). "Me time" is important to our well being. Boundaries are another part of self love. If we allow others to overstep their reach, they can take away our power to be who we are. Don't be afraid to say "no" or to take action to preserve your self respect, dignity, and personal needs.

My fix, along with the clarity of vision, told me I needed to take some action toward reconnecting with my soul, spirit, God, and my vision for my purpose and destiny. Like the surgery for my eye, I needed to see my path clearly again. This "reconnection" would assist in that. My dreams—my vision—had been like a map to guide me forward. Slowly its ideal, like my physical sight, had been fading away. I'd allowed its guidance to become disconnected. I needed a fix to regain the clarity I'd once had.

Earlier, I asked, what changes were forced upon you because of your ailment? I found myself forced into resting mode. The quiet contemplation, meditation-like state required after my surgery, helped me reconnect to my eternal self. (Who says ailments are bad when they are so powerful to realign us?)

Thus, I know that this step is one meant for me to take, necessary not just for the healing of my eye, but for the reconnection and healing of my life. (Notice how the word "reconnection" sneaks in there, while it is also associated with the ailment itself.)

As a side note, my eye surgeon prescribed drops designed to "lower the pressure" in my eye. It would not be a stretch to say I needed to lower the self pressure on myself. Answers to our forward path are all around us, if we are open to seeing them.

Sometimes the fix is something obvious that you knew you *should be* doing but weren't. I've had clients leave jobs they have wanted to exit from for years. One client decided to have some surgery he'd been putting off; it changed his life in magical ways. One client finally bought the house of her dreams. Others have left crumbling relationships they struggled with for too long.

Ultimately, your fix should conclude with one clear focus. By finding your personal meaning, your action steps should create joy and lead you toward fulfilling the desires of your heart. Your symptoms, when looked at through a deeper lens, are merely providing intuitive guidance to help you do so.

After You've Created a Viable "Fix"

Your next step is to *implement* the Guided Action Step you've intuited. This step may require bold action or a gradual, methodical change. It may require planning. You may also need to consider additional symptoms (if they are occurring), and *their* message, which could add further insights.

Everybody's situation and "fix" are different. Typically, I find that my clients already knew about the problem showing up through this affliction. They may have even known what steps they needed to take—but hadn't. Taking those steps may feel scary, uncertain, or life-complicating. Sometimes it seems easier to simply be in pain. But believe me, it's not.

Always keep in mind that if you haven't acted on your created Guided Action Step, it might be because you think it's too hard or too complicated, yet your body is saying, *"There is a way!"*

I often remember author Carol Adrienne saying, *"If you are having a hard time choosing between two different options, there might be a third option you haven't thought of yet."*

Sometimes we get so focused on what we *think* the answer is, we overlook some other answer that is easier and more beneficial for everyone involved. Other times, we are so focused on the journey to the resolution, we forget it's okay to simply take one step at a time. Take that first step, then decide on the next and the next.

It is often this challenging, forward step that helps propel us into a more fulfilling life. When I had cancer in my 20s, I had no clue it would one day lead to me being an author and healer. I knew my illness was challenging me to stand up for myself and to take charge of my life. I had to learn to voice my opinions and speak up for my beliefs. It wasn't always easy to do that. I worried about how the people in my life might react. But if I hadn't taken those steps, who knows where would I be today.

If you're unable to create the necessary resolution because it involves a person who has died or is no longer in contact with you—and there is no way for that to change—instead, *visualize* a happy resolution. See the appropriate support people or resources coming in for this person. See it resolved. The brain (or body) can't tell the difference as long as it is a visceral experience.

Remember, you must apply the Guided Action Step for a shift to take place in your life. When you *do* apply it, you will see changes occur, often more quickly than you expected.

Use the following page to write out your Guided Action Step(s). Include how and when you will take these actions.

Write your Guided Action Step in the box below:

If You're Still Unsure About the "Fix"

If your Guided Action Step feels weak, unclear, or impossible to implement, try having a friend help you. See what insights your friend might offer, as they can often see obvious connections in your life you're overlooking because you're too close to it.

Go back once more to review your mechanic's story, your x-ray, and your fix. Are there any areas you can better clarify with different words or different meanings for those words? Have you left out anything important? Have you made your description too generic?

I've had clients tell me "I don't have any symptoms," but as we start talking, they will admit, "I do get sinus headaches," or "I do have a sore knee," or something of the like. For whatever reason, they either discounted the symptom, forgot about it, or simply didn't feel comfortable revealing it at the start.

Still stuck? Would you like a little more help? Do you crave a deeper insight? You can send your collection of findings to me for review and assessment!

Visit this special, for my readers only web page for your options. This offer has limited availability, so don't delay!

https://tinyurl.com/yc3jkxyt

Appendix

We must be right in heart and head today
in order to secure a happy tomorrow.
Do what is right under the circumstances.
Do your best!
Be certain that your still small voice—
the angel of your heart—
approves of what you do.

Andrew Jackson Davis
The Great Harmonia, Vol. 3, p. 362

More Healing Steps

After I create my imaginary fix, I take time to visualize healing light and energy flowing into my body to repair whatever might have occurred there.

It's never a good idea to overthink a symptom. Always release it when done and "see" it as healed.

Golden, Sparkly Goo

Reverend Shirley Caulkins Smith, who spent her last years living in the spiritual community of Lily Dale, NY, taught us to visualize "golden, sparkling goo" flowing down from the heavens into our body. Allow it to flow through, touch, and heal everything within you.

The Energy Ball

Our hands carry and transmit energy. You can rub your hands together until you feel warmth. Then hold one or both hands over the area to be healed. If you hold them just an inch or so from your body you may feel heat or other energies entering into the area. Accept the healing you are receiving and offer thanks.

Also look for my book: *Marvelous Messages from Your Faith,* in which I share effective use of prayers.

Body Image

I've often experimented using this process with my body image—specifically, weight gain and areas of excess fat. While not perfected *(meaning, it hasn't caused me to lose weight or fat—yet)*, here are some tips if you want to try it.

> ▷ Hone in on a particular area (i.e., belly, hips, upper arms, etc.).

> ▷ Follow the method protocols to gather keywords, meanings, and your deeper life connections.

> ▷ Speak to the chosen body part as if it's part of your Inner Child, asking him/her how s/he feels and what s/he needs. (These needs are your points of action.) You may find these statements encompass several "symptoms" or needs, each requiring separate evaluation.

> ▷ The ancestral connection may also be a key factor here, especially with relatives who lived through famine or tremendous stress. Looking at photographs can provide clues to their physique.

> ▷ The fix is rarely anything to do with diets, calories, exercise, or other common weight loss myths, but will likely begin with you addressing your underlying emotional needs. For example, I often am "carrying extra weight" when I take on too much in my daily life.

Innate Challenges

An *innate challenge* is an inborn struggle we face, often multiple times throughout our lives, as a part of our spiritual evolution.

Whether we recognize it or not, we are constantly replicating the challenges faced by our ancestors. Some of their challenges, in a personal and unique way, show up as our challenges. (These seem to be dealt randomly to the family like a deck of cards.)

I like to compare it to flowers. A gardener plants some daisies. Perhaps they grow under normal conditions and are beautiful. He gathers the seeds and passes some to a friend. Perhaps the friend plants the seeds, but not in good soil, or maybe she doesn't water them enough. The new flowers grow, produce seeds, but these seeds remember their adverse growing conditions. They encode themselves with that memory. They may form a defense mechanism for when they regenerate (humans call this a *survival strategy*). Thus, the environment the daisies are subjected to greatly affects themselves and their progeny.

I've seen that the more I take notice of and confront these challenges, the more I move ahead toward my soul's calling. The first step in doing so is simply to recognize them when they occur. The second is choosing how we *react* to them. Often, it's simply a case of rewriting old family paradigms, something we may be doing as a natural part of who we are. This all comes back to our physical body and the messages it's sending us. It remembers our past and the past that came before us.

Ancestral Healing

If you'd like to take the Marvelous Messages process deeper, I recommend you explore your ancestry and innate challenges further. Here's how I do that.

First, I select an ancestor from my bloodline. Although it doesn't matter how far back I go, I must know of an illness they suffered from or how they died. At times, I have found this through archived newspaper articles or by viewing death certificates found on ancestry search sites.

Once I know this information, I begin to use the same process detailed in this book, with the difference that the fix can no longer help them and the challenges they faced but can, instead, be perceived as a gift they pass to me to help me face mine.

However, I am looking at this purely as a means to better understand my own innate challenges, and from the perspective that it is all speculative. As long as I keep that in mind, it is a fun process that offers me some interesting insights.

I've also discussed this process in my book *Hatch – A Change Your Life Guide*, or watch for my forthcoming book and card deck: *Marvelous Messages from Your Ancestry*.

Mirrors

Earlier, I mentioned "mirrors" and how we sometimes find a "coincidental" occurrence of a particular symptom or ailment showing up in and around our lives.

Your co-worker arrives Monday morning with a broken leg; you watch a movie, and the hero has a broken leg; you go to the doctor and hold the door open for a women with a broken leg. "What's up with all these broken legs?" you wonder.

This is often a good time to ask yourself, "what's broken in my life?" or do a quick analysis on any keywords that come up for you in association with "broken," "legs," or other connections. Are you about to suffer a broken leg yourself? (I hope not!) But be aware of "coincidental" happenings in your life. You can often extract meaning and direction from them without having to suffer yourself.

A Favor?

Can I ask a favor? If you enjoyed *Marvelous Messages from Your Body* it would mean a lot if you would let your friends know so they can also experience these ideas. Most social and retail platforms make it easy to click and share.

If you leave a review for the book on the site from which you purchased it, on Goodreads, your own blog, or your favorite social media platform, I would love to read it. Tag me, or email me the link at **info@saloff.com**.

I would also enjoy hearing about your experiences using any part of my Marvelous Messages™ process. Email me or feel free to post your questions and comments on my website or any of my social media platforms (links are in my bio at the end of the book). Your valuable feedback helps me to evolve my systems so they can better help others.

Next Steps

The Marvelous Messages process is comprised of five levels: the Heart, the Root (your heritage), Connection (to the Divine), Overcoming Obstacles (blocking your way), and Transformation (ascension—or more precisely, achieving that "happy place" you've sought for so long). *Marvelous Messages from Your Body* is part of the Heart level.

I recommend you explore the Heart level first, as this will lead you to all else you desire. The Heart level books include this work, *Marvelous Messages from Your Childhood,* and my forthcoming book, *Marvelous Messages from Your Heart.*

Next, I recommend exploring your roots, as you will uncover some of the innate challenges ingrained within you and the means to overcome them. I explain this in my book, *Hatch – A Change Your Life Guide,* or watch for my forthcoming book *Marvelous Messages from Your Ancestry* and its accompanying card deck for more hands-on guidance.

The exercises in this book describe the **quickie** method for the Heart level of the Marvelous Messages process. If you are having a hard time seeing the fix or discovering your Guided Action Step, personalized coaching may help you to go deeper into the layers of your symptoms.

In private coaching with me, we work together through this process to reveal your innate challenges and free your most heartfelt desires. I use my intuitive abilities to part the veil and connect with your ancestry. We explore your challenges, desires, and their core essence on multiple levels. Visit my website to learn more.

In addition, you might consider any of the following options:

▷ Watch for additional *Marvelous Messages* books coming soon.

▷ Visit my website for additional articles, audios, videos, resource links, and other materials designed to help you utilize your Marvelous Messages.

▷ Watch for my interactive classes and coaching.

▷ Check for my Facebook groups and connect with me via social media.

If you're ready to experience more, visit my website at:

www.MarvelousMessages.com

About Jamie Linn Saloff

Author, teacher, story weaver, spiritual counselor, seer of visions, pathfinder. . . for over thirty years Jamie has taught type-A-driven free spirits how to become happy, healthy, and wealthy by listening to their body groan and their soul weep.

Jamie strongly believes in the inherent power of our ancestry and in *"looking back to leap forward."* She has frequently appeared as a radio personality, guest blogger, and workshop leader. She has written and been featured in countless articles, blogs, newsletters, and newspapers. Jamie has authored twelve books including:

▷ *Hatch – A Change Your Life Guide*

▷ *Marvelous Messages from Your Childhood*: Thirteen Traits that Reveal Your Hidden Potential and Empower You to Answer the Calling of Your Heart

▷ *Marvelous Messages from Your Faith*: A Simple and Effective Method to Manifest Your Desires and Receive More Answers to Your Prayers

▷ Be sure to watch for other forthcoming works in the Marvelous Messages series of books, including *Marvelous Messages from Your Ancestry* and its accompanying card deck.

View her books on Amazon here: https://amzn.to/3s837aJ

Jamie has trained with many professional practitioners, healers, and coaches including Elaine and Mark Thomas, Tom Cratsley, Donna Eden, Bill Coller, Lisa Williams, Shirley Caulkins Smith, Sharon Klingler, Sig Longren, Joey Korn, Daniel Hardt, (and many more). She is certified Reiki I. She is a minister and multi-certified graduate of Lily Dale's Fellowships of the Spirit.

In her free time, Jamie enjoys needlecrafts, making jewelry, and golf. She spends time studying spirituality, metaphysics, and parapsychology. She is a Mac geek and spends way too much time on the computer. She lives in PA and NY with her husband and a very spoiled cat. She has two grown sons.

Follow Jamie on the web at:

▷ **Website:** www.MarvelousMessages.com
   (Receive a free gift when you stop by)

▷ **Facebook:** www.facebook.com/JamieLSaloff

▷ **Instagram**: www.instagram.com/jamie_saloff

▷ **Twitter:** http://twitter.com/JamieSaloff

▷ **Linkedin:** www.linkedin.com/in/jamiesaloff

—␣—

What Others Are Saying About Jamie

"My session with Jamie felt like a FASCINATING journey through my body and my issues with chronic pain. She provided me with great insight as to how to move forward in the healing process, and how to "lighten my load." I seriously had one "Ah-ha" moment after another! After our session ended, I sat quietly contemplating what had been revealed to me through Jamie, and I felt totally empowered to take action in finding the balance needed to heal certain areas of my life. I highly recommend working with Jamie!"

~ Joy Phillips, OnceUponAnArchetype.com

"Jamie does something that is very wonderful. When I started talking with her I felt like I was stuck in a dark forest and did not know which way to turn. Jamie very calmly started asking me questions and making some great connections based on what I was telling her. She took me through the bushes and brambles and lead me into the light. I am now moving forward in the direction that is right for me. Thanks, Jamie, You Rock!"

~ LeeAnn Putnam

"Jamie Saloff is an amazing coach! Her insight and intuition mean she has the incredible ability to get to the heart of the matter quickly and come up with workable practical solutions just as quickly. I was struggling with a thorny personal issue and within just one hour Jamie helped me feel lighter, happier and I knew the clear path to resolve the issue. Easy as pie! If you need help sorting out some of the challenges you face—not just a person to vent to—but someone who will help you arrive at real, workable solutions, contact her today! Thanks, Jamie."

~ Denise Michaels, Las Vegas, NV, DeniseMichaels.com

I am grateful to Jamie for her intuitive listening skills and her ability to help me to understand how my body is telling where to focus attention on my life's journey. Her guidance as a medium brought phenomenal comfort to me. I applaud Jamie's skills and appreciate the knowledge, compassion, and excitement she brings to each session. She is a helper, a healer, and a conduit of messages.

~ Carolyn Hilsdon Gilles

Notes

www.ingramcontent.com/pod-product-compliance
Lightning Source LLC
Chambersburg PA
CBHW071124030426
42336CB00013BA/2194